How to Design and Finance Workplace Health Promotion Programs

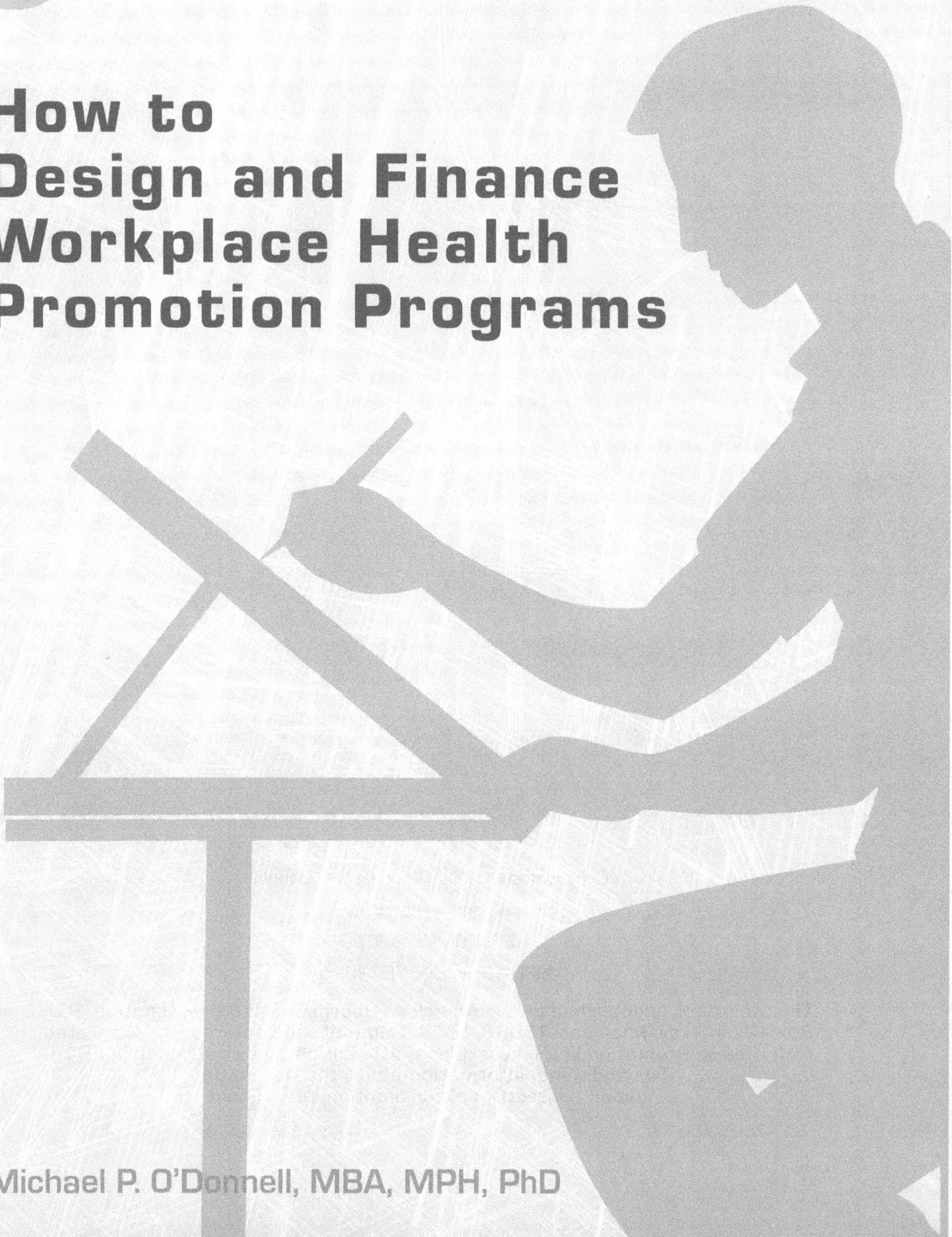

Michael P. O'Donnell, MBA, MPH, PhD

This workbook is published by the American Journal of Health Promotion. P.O. Box 1254, Troy, Michigan 48099-1254. Some of the contents are excerpted from Health Promotion in the Workplace, 4th Edition, to be published in 2014. For additional information about the 4th Edition e-mail contact@healthpromotionjournal.com.

How to Design and Finance Workplace Health Promotion Programs

Michael P. O'Donnell, MBA, MPH, PhD

AMERICAN JOURNAL *of*

Health Promotion

Table of Contents

INTRODUCTION

The purpose of this workbook is to describe a process that can be used by any employer or consultant to design a workplace health promotion program. It incorporates the AMSO Framework and draws on the definition of health promotion articulated by the *American Journal of Health Promotion*[1] (See Table 1). The process also reflects the findings of a benchmarking study conducted by the author on the best workplace health promotion programs.[2]

Table 1

Definition of Health Promotion

"Health Promotion is the art and science of helping people discover the synergies between their core passions and optimal health, enhancing their motivation to strive for optimal health, and supporting them in changing their lifestyle to move toward a state of optimal health. Optimal health is a dynamic balance of physical, emotional, social, spiritual, and intellectual health. Lifestyle change can be facilitated through a combination of learning experiences that enhance awareness, increase motivation, and build skills and, most important, through the creation of opportunities that open access to environments that make positive health practices the easiest choice."

Source: M. O'Donnell, *American Journal of Health Promotion,* 2009

The goal of that study was to identify the best ***workplace health promotion programs*** in the United States and determine what made them different from the hundreds of other programs in place. The eight elements unique to these programs are shown in Table 2. These elements are organized in a matrix in terms of the impact of the element on program outcome and the level of control a typical program manager would have over building that element into their program. For example, linking the goals of the program to the business goals of the organization has a major impact on the effectiveness of the program and is also something the typical program manager can control. The manager can articulate the goals of the organization and align the program goals to support these organization goals. Not surprisingly, another factor that was very important in determining the success of the program was strong top management support. Unfortunately, in the short term, the typical program manager has little control over how much support they receive from top management. Interestingly, having a large program budget was only moderately important in determining the success of a program. Most of the programs studied did have generous budgets, but many of the programs not deemed among the "best" also had strong program budgets. A strong program budget is important, but it is not sufficient to make a program successful.

Table 2

Characteristics of Best Workplace Health Promotion Programs

	Low Impact	Medium Impact	High Impact
High Control		• effective communicaton • communicate evaluation results	• link programs to business goals
Medium Control		• evaluation component	• incentive program
Low Control		• strong budget	• supportive culture • top management support

The striking finding of this study was that management-related factors were more important than programming factors in determining the success of the program. The typical health promotion program manager who is trained as a health expert tends to focus on the health dimensions of a program and often neglects how the program ties into the organization. A team putting together a new health promotion program should build each of these eight qualities into their new program.

The design process described here has three basic stages: preparing for the design process, collecting data and determining the program content and management structure for the program.

PHASE I: STRUCTURING THE DESIGN PROCESS

The design process described here is fairly elaborate and participatory. It assumes that the organization is starting at the beginning, not yet having decided even whether it is ready to develop a health promotion program. Each organization will have to adapt this process to meet its specific situation and the protocols it normally follows to develop a program.

Before an organization starts the design process, it should prepare for the design process by answering four basic questions:

1. How ready is the organization to develop a health promotion program?
2. Are the program outcome expectations realistic?
3. How participative a process does the organization want to follow in designing the program?
4. How extensive a design process does it wish to follow?

Each of these questions is discussed in the paragraphs that follow.

Stages of Readiness

Table 3 shows the various **stages of readiness** in which an organization might find itself and the action it should take for that level of readiness. This is not an exhaustive list of stages, but it covers the full range of situations.

Table 3

Stages of Organizational Readiness

Stage	Action
Not interested	Sell the concept or wait
Interested in concept but not sure if it will work	Conduct feasibility study
Sold on concept	Conduct needs assessment
Impatient for program	Implement quickly

At one extreme, an analyst or program proponent might find that the organization or key decision makers are not at all interested in health promotion. Starting a design process would be a waste of time. Although a **feasibility study** might uncover some good financial arguments for the program and some pockets of support, it would probably not be taken seriously if no interest exists and would be difficult to complete without a fair degree of cooperation. The analyst or proponent could probably best use his or her time selling the concept.

In another case, the decision makers might be totally sold on the concept and committed to developing a program, but, because of lack of knowledge of program options and benefits, employees might have little interest in the programs. The proponent might de-emphasize the cost/benefit part of the research and follow a design process committed to heavy employee participation.

In some companies, extensive research on feasibility and employee interests may have been completed, and the desired program has been outlined. Collecting extensive additional data and taking months to analyze it might exhaust the patience of the leadership and allow excitement to develop a program to dissipate. The effort might be most successful if it bypasses much of the research and design phases described here and proceeds directly to implementation.

Finally, if the organization is committed to developing a program but resources are inadequate to develop a comprehensive one, the program designer might do additional research to establish the need and secure the resources for a more comprehensive program.

Each organization should determine its stage of readiness within the continuum shown in Table 3 and enter the design process at the appropriate stage.

Setting Realistic Goals

As a discipline, workplace health promotion is in the mid-adolescent stage. Some significant programs have been in place for almost 50 years, and the vast majority of large workplaces have some form of program.[3] Health promotion programs are found in all types of large and small, white- and blue-collar, public and private sector organizations. As a science, health promotion is pushing from its late childhood to early adolescence. Major teaching institutions offer health promotion majors; major research institutions are involved in health promotion; thousands of studies have been published on the health impact of programs; behavior change theory is finally being translated into practical applications and health promotion concepts have been integrated into national policy. In clinical settings, intensive health promotion techniques have even been able to reduce heart disease.[4] Despite this progress, the science of workplace health promotion still has many limits. In fact, as our science has improved, the limits of our current programs become more clear.

It *is* realistic to

- Engage a large portion of employees in programs
- Help a significant portion of participants to improve in some areas, including
    - Quit smoking
    - Reduce dietary fat consumption
    - Reduce blood pressure
    - Reduce cholesterol
    - Reduce absenteeism
    - Increase seat belt use
    - Increase levels of physical activity
    - Reduce heavy alcohol use
    - Reduce medical costs
    - Learn how to better manage stress

It *may not* be realistic to see a substantial number of employees

- Lose weight
- Improve fitness
- Increase fruit and vegetable consumption

It is *not* realistic to:

- Expect no relapses to past poor health behaviors
- Reverse significantly deteriorated health conditions in less than five years
- Expect major improvements in health conditions without major effort
- Expect health improvements to continue after a program is discontinued

It is also *not* realistic to:

- Expect 100% participation in programs
- See major reduction in health care expenditures within a few years without major investments in the programs
- See increased job output from all participants in the program

As we perfect our methods, improve our diffusion of knowledge among health promotion professionals, and perfect our execution, we should expect lower relapse rates, greater success in reversing significantly deteriorated health conditions, and higher participation rates in programs. We should never expect major payoffs to the sponsoring organization without a significant investment of resources.

The program developer must also be assertive, yet realistic about getting clarification on what top management will agree to in the design and implementation of the program. The developer should be assertive by insisting that health promotion be treated as an investment that will benefit the organization, not as an extravagant benefit for employees that can be cut when money is short. The organization may discover through the health promotion program that it should enhance some of its communication practices, refine its organization structure, or do a better job of involving employees in its decision making. Although the need for these changes might be recognized as a result of the health promotion program, they are changes that will ultimately facilitate the organization's basic goals.

Major shifts that benefit the health promotion program but detract from the organization's basic mission or clash with its culture should not be expected. For example, allowing employees flextime or time off work to participate in programs might have a significant impact on success of the program but may be impractical in many organizations. Flexible (or cafeteria) benefits may generate funds for the health promotion program by allowing employees to apply some of their benefit dollars to programs. However, if the cost of developing and managing a flexible benefit program is greater than the projected benefits of the health promotion program, it has little chance of being implemented.

The ultimate corporate goal of the health promotion program is to make the organization better able to achieve its strategic goals. Therefore the health promotion program must be molded to fit the organization. The organization will not be molded to fit the health promotion program.

Table 4 shows the likelihood of achieving various organization goals with each of the different levels of programs. For example, the table suggests it is unlikely that an awareness program will reduce medical care costs but it is probable that a program that utilizes all four elements of the **AMSO Framework** will reduce medical care costs. This table will help the design team and management set realistic goals for the program. The typical struggle occurs when top management wants to achieve a wide range of ambitious organization goals but wants to invest a small amount of money. This chart helps them realize significant programs will be required to achieve significant organization goals. If there is a mismatch between goals and budget, one of the two must change. This table should be used during the initial planning stages and later in the process when actual program content is being developed.

Table 4

Impact of Program Levels on Achieving Organization Goals

Organization Goals	Level I Awareness Only	Level II 2-3 AMSO Elements	Level III 4 AMSO Elements
Enhance Image			
General visibility	unlikely	maybe	very probable
Recruiting	maybe	maybe	very probable
Institutional relationships	unlikely	maybe	maybe
Related product image	unlikely	maybe	probable
Enhance Productivity			
Morale	probable	probable	very probable
Turnover	unlikely	maybe	very probable

Table 4 continued

Absenteeism	maybe	probable	very probable
Physical stamina	unlikely	probable	probable
Emotional hardiness	unlikely	maybe	probable
Desire to work	maybe	maybe	very probable
Reduce Medically Related Costs			
Medical crises	unlikely	maybe	probable
Medical premiums	maybe	probable	very probable
Disability costs	maybe	probable	very probable
Workers compensation costs	maybe	maybe	probable
Life insurance	unlikely	maybe	maybe

Employee Involvement in the Design Process

Participation by employees in the design process is essential to the success of the program. Employees must know that the program is designed to meet *their* needs and that *their* involvement is critical to the success of the program.

The degree of employee involvement in the design process for the health promotion process should be significant in all organizations but should fall within the range of employee involvement in other comparable decision processes in that organization. The range of participation levels is listed in Table 5.

Table 5

Degree of Employee Participation in the Design Process

1. Top management directs process and makes all decisions
2. Top management directs process and makes all decisions but seeks input
3. Top management retains decision making but shares direction of process
4. Top management shares decision making and direction of process
5. Employees direct process and decision making

The employees' level of authority within this design process might be further defined or limited to developing components of the program. For example, top management might have authority to set financial budgets; a consultant or subject-matter expert might have authority to determine specific curriculum and protocols; and the employees on the design committee might have authority to determine specific topics, program components, types of promotional efforts, and operational protocols.

Employee Committee

An **Employee Health Promotion Committee** can provide a very effective mechanism to ensure employee involvement in the design process. The committee will probably be most effective and efficient if it has at least six and no more than sixteen members, representing the types of employees listed here.

- Top management spokesperson
- Health benefits manager
- Education and training manager
- Recreation programs coordinator
- Recruiting employment manager
- Medical department coordinator
- Employee association(s) representative
- Union representative(s) (if a large portion of employees is represented by unions)
- Employee(s)-at-large representing various departments
- Middle management representative(s)
- Facilitator
- Communication manager
- Technical expert

A smaller committee is easier to manage; a larger committee may provide better representation of important interest groups.

Committees provide an excellent mechanism for involving employees in decision making, for generating ideas, and for stimulating input from many interest groups. Committees can also be very time-consuming and get bogged down in the decision making process. Committees will be most effective if their purpose and degree of authority in each area covered is clearly stated and if they are coordinated by an experienced facilitator. Table 6 shows the topics of meetings of an actual committee in which the participation level (from Table 5) was "Top management shares decision making and direction of the process with employees."

Table 6

Topics of Meetings in Typical Design Process

Meeting Number	Topics Covered at Meeting
1	Stimulus for program Role and process clarification Education on health promotion
2	Education on health promotion Presentation of data collected to date
3	Education on health promotion Data collection plan
4	Report on data collection findings
5	Synthesis: Organization and health improvement goals
6	Synthesis: Program content and administrative structure
7	Discussion of proposal 1st draft
8	Discussion of proposal 2nd draft
9	Ratification of 3rd draft to be sent to top management

Knowledge and Expertise Required to Design a Health Promotion Program

Employees on the committee should be given authority to set goals and policies to the extent approved by the organization. They should be involved in selecting program topics and developing program protocols, but they should be careful not to exceed their level of knowledge and skill in clinical and organizational areas of health promotion. The individuals responsible for designing the program should have expertise in all of the following areas:

- Organizational theory
- Group process
- Operations management
- Communication and marketing methods
- Motivation techniques
- Design process

- Clinical aspects of health promotion, including
  - health assessment
  - fitness
  - nutrition
  - stress management
  - smoking cessation
  - medical self-care
  - social health

Few organizations will have all of these knowledge areas represented within their existing staff. They can develop or acquire knowledge in these areas by educating existing staff, hiring new staff members with the necessary knowledge, or working with a consultant.

Magnitude of the Design Process

An extensive design process will not be necessary for all organizations. Organizations that have already completed some phases of the process described above can skip those stages. Organizations that know ahead of time that they want a very simple program do not need an extensive process. Organizations working with external vendors can sometimes rely on the vendor's expertise and shorten some of the steps. Each organization must determine the extent of the process appropriate for its needs but err on the side of a more extensive process. The process described here is probably most appropriate for an organization with 4,000-10,000 employees. Smaller or larger employers or those developing less-comprehensive programs can follow the same framework but adjust the magnitude of the design process accordingly.

Extra time and resources spent on collecting data will provide additional baseline data for later measures of program success. Extra time and resources spent in the design process will increase the opportunity for employee involvement and the likelihood of an appropriate design. Extra time and resources spent on implementation will increase the chances of having a program that is introduced effectively. A surprisingly large number of employers simplify this process and rely on vendors for guidance on many of the issues described here. While this saves significant time in the short run, it reduces the employer's understanding of the intricacies of the program and increases the employer's dependence on the vendor.

Developing and implementing a health promotion program in moderate- to large-sized organizations normally takes 6 to 18 months but can sometimes take years. The typical development timetable is shown in Table 7. The time can be on the short side if management is committed to moving quickly

10

and resources are available to design and implement a program. The timetable can be compressed significantly if pressure to reduce medical care costs is severe, or if an outside group, like the health insurance vendor, implements a turnkey program. In many cases, however, there is a longer period of "gestation" in which management is becoming familiar with the health promotion concept and is not yet ready to develop a program. In general, the process takes longer in larger organizations, especially if data is required from multiple locations, multiple levels of approval are required, and programs are implemented over time at different locations.

Table 7

Development Timetable

Stage of Development	Timetable
Gestation	0-24 months
Assessment	2-12 months
Design	2-12 months
Approval	1-12 months
Implementation	3-36 months

PHASE II: COLLECTING DATA – CONDUCTING A FEASIBILITY STUDY OR NEEDS ASSESSMENT

The second major step in the design process is collecting data to gather the information necessary to design the program. This can take the form of a **feasibility study** or a **needs assessment**. In some instances, the data collection may be designed to determine if the organization should or should not develop a program. In these cases the data collection might be called a "feasibility study." In other circumstances the decision to develop the program may have already been made, and the data collection may be designed to determine how the program should be developed. This data collection might be called a "needs assessment."

The specific focus and the use of the information derived from these two types of studies will be slightly different, but the tools and process used for both will be very much the same. Moreover, a comprehensive feasibility study can answer both whether or not a program should be developed and how it should be developed. Organizations that have already decided to develop a program can make slight adaptions to this approach in data collection.

If an organization expects to evaluate the effectiveness of its program in achieving stated goals, it should expect to collect some data in addition to the basic data collected for the feasibility study.

The feasibility study answers the basic question: Is it feasible for this organization to develop and operate a health promotion program? Five specific questions are addressed in dealing with this basic issue:

1. What are the organization's goals and motives for considering the development of a program?
2. Is a health promotion program a cost-effective investment for this organization?
3. What are the levels of support, need, and interest among employees, middle managers, and top managers?
4. Does the organization have access to the necessary resources within the organization and the community?

If the answers to the first four questions indicate that the program is feasible, the last question is:

5. What are the key factors that should be considered during the actual program design process?

In addition to answering the basic feasibility questions, this study provides much of the background information required for the design process and provides an opportunity to promote the health promotion program among many of the people who will be crucial to its success. It also provides much of the baseline data against which future progress can be measured.

The time and other resources spent on the feasibility study should be determined by the quality of information required and by the impact of that information on the eventual design process. A basic study will take an experienced analyst 40-120 hours over 4-16 weeks if needed data is readily available. If the study is for a large organization, if data are not available, if a major investment needs to be made in the program, or if there is significant controversy surrounding the prospect of a program, the study can take far more time.

Clarification of Motives and Goals

"We want to have a health promotion program. Let's design one like XYZ Company. The program can reduce our medical care costs, enhance our image, and improve our productivity." This is the typical summary of an employer explaining the concept of and goals for a health promotion program. Unfortunately, if the concept and goals are not further clarified before a program is developed, achieving any of the stated benefits will be almost entirely coincidental.

To be successful, the employer's position should be rephrased. "We want to reduce medical care costs, improve our productivity, and enhance our image. We will develop a health promotion program designed to achieve these goals." With this approach, the employer decides which benefits are most important and then designs a program specifically to achieve them.

It is all right for the organization to:

- Think the health promotion concept makes sense and, therefore, to want to develop a program.
- Be altruistic and want to improve the well-being of its employees by sponsoring a health promotion program.
- Expand the goals of the program after it has had more experience with the program and better understands the potential benefits.

However, in designing the programs, the goals must be clarified and the design process must be directed by the goals. If not, there is much less chance the program will benefit the organization. Major problems in the mismatch of design and goals occur for the following reasons:

- Most managers and executives don't know enough about health promotion programs to realize the time required for the design process.
- Most health promotion program designers don't understand organizations well enough to know the range of benefits that may result from the programs—nor do they understand program design or health promotion well enough to design the program to achieve specific goals.
- Most health promotion program designers don't understand group process well enough to help the organization articulate the goals for the program.
- Many organizations don't adequately clarify the goals of any of their activities.

If the goals of the program are going to be adequately clarified, significant effort will be required to direct the goal clarification process. This will include convincing top management that goal clarification sessions are necessary. The extent of the goal clarification process and the overall program design process will, of course, depend on the extent of the program to be designed.

Most of the goals of the program can be categorized under two headings: **management goals** and **health goals**. Management goals will include reduction in medical care costs, enhanced image, and improved productivity. Health goals will address the level of health change desired and the specific *area* of change, such as nutrition or fitness. Management and health goals will not always be achieved through the same program design, and the relative priorities of the two will certainly impact the focus of the program.

For example, if the management goal of reducing medical care costs were the primary goal, the following process might be followed:

1. Analyze past, current, and projected health care expenditures for patterns and high-cost areas.
2. Determine current and projected future health conditions of employees as they relate to health care expenditures. This is done through health screenings and by reviewing medical insurance and worker's compensation records.
3. Determine which health conditions have the greatest impact on cost and which can be successfully addressed by health promotion programs.
4. Perform a cost/benefit analysis to determine which programs produce benefits that are greater than their cost.
5. Investigate methods to correct or prevent the high-cost health conditions that cannot be affected by health promotion.
6. Develop methods to track the impact of the program on health care costs.
7. Develop health promotion programs that will have the greatest impact on medical care costs. These will probably include special programs for employees with the highest medical care costs, smoking cessation, hypertension control, prevention of lower back problems, auto safety, and general injury prevention programs.

If the goal is a health goal, such as reducing the incidence of heart attacks, the following very different process might be followed:

1. Determine causes of heart attacks.
2. Determine which of these causes can be affected by health promotion programs.
3. Conduct screening of employees to identify cardiac risk factors.
4. Determine which programs are most effective in reducing the cardiac risk factors in the employee population.
5. Investigate methods to correct the cardiac risk factors that cannot be reduced by the health promotion program.
6. Develop methods to track the impact of the programs on cardiac risk factors.
7. Develop the programs that will have the greatest impact on cardiac risk factors. These will probably include nutrition, smoking cessation, fitness, stress management, hypertension control, and social support enhancement.

If the goal is a management goal to enhance the image of the organization, the following process might be followed:

1. Determine the groups and individuals whose perception of the organization is most important.
2. Determine the components of a health promotion program most likely to shape this group's perception and develop these programs.
3. Develop mechanisms to capitalize on the image value of the program.
4. Investigate methods to enhance image other than the health promotion program.
5. Develop methods to track the impact of the program on image.
6. Develop other non-health promotion programs that will have the greatest impact on image.

In most cases there will be multiple goals. The challenge to the program designer is to accurately determine the relative priorities of the goals and to design the program to achieve the appropriate balance of benefits in each of the goal areas.

In virtually every case, a third major consideration – in addition to the health and organization goals – will be limits on the human, financial, spatial, and time resources available for the program. These will limit the range of program options considered and will force the programs to be designed in such a way that they achieve the greatest possible return on investment.

The importance of clarifying motives and goals is illustrated by the results of the benchmarking study. The most successful programs tied their program goals to the organization's goals. If the goals are not clarified, the goals cannot be aligned.

It is often difficult for an organization to clarify the goals of a proposed health promotion program. This is true because most executives do not have a precise understanding of the potential benefits of a health promotion program. Also, all large organizations are composed of many decision makers or top managers. It would not be unusual for one manager to expect the health promotion program to reduce medical care costs by 15 percent and another manager within the same organization to expect the program to have no impact on medical care costs. One solution to this problem is to have a clear protocol for clarifying goals. The five-step process outlined here has been used effectively by a number of organizations to clarify goals.

Cost/Benefit Analysis Projections

Like any other program in the organization, the health promotion program should not be a frill. It should pay for itself in terms of the benefits it brings to the organization. Some of these benefits will be tangible and measurable, such as reduced medical care costs or reduced absentee-ism. Others will be more difficult to measure but equally valuable, such as improved image. Projecting the financial returns a program may generate is not simple, but it can and should be done as part of the feasibility study to determine if the program is a good investment for the organization.

Levels of Support and Areas of Interest

Broad-based and strong support among all levels of employees is critical to the success of the health promotion program. Measuring the level of support during the research phase will show how support figures into the overall design strategy. If support is very strong, that alone may be enough to convince those in power that a program should be developed. If support is very weak but all other measures in the feasibility study indicate that a health promotion program makes sense, program designers should be prepared to allocate a significant portion of resources to promotion of the pro-gram. Support should be measured at three levels:

1. Top management
2. Middle management
3. General employee population

Support at all levels is important, but support from top management is probably the most im-portant if the program is going to get off the ground. This support means much more than just agreeing with the concept of the program. Positive answers to all of the following questions show strong support. For example, will top management agree to the following:

- Will they act as a role model by participating in the program?
- Will they promote the program regularly through formal and informal statements of support?
- Will they provide financial backing for the program?
- Will they provide administrative support through facilities maintenance, financial access to com-munication channels, and effective supervision?
- Will they be open to reviewing and possibly changing policies that do not encourage a healthy lifestyle?

Table 8 shows a more detailed set of questions that can be used in structured interviews with top managers. These interviews will also provide an opportunity to articulate the mission, long-term goals, and current priorities of the organization.

Table 8

Questions to Ask Top Managers

1. Program Content
    - What is your concept of a health promotion program?
    - What kinds of programs would work best for this organization?
    - What level of programs (awareness, behavior change, supportive environments) makes the most sense for this organization?

2. Support
    - Would you personally participate in the program?
    - Would you encourage the managers who report to you to participate in the program and to encourage their employees to participate?
    - Would you be available to help in promoting the program to employees in general?
    - Would you be available to troubleshoot if the program needs help?
    - How strong do you expect support for the program to be at each level of the organization?

3. Benefits
    - What do you see as the qualitative and quantitative benefits of a health promotion program for this organization? What percentage improvements would you see in medical care costs and productivity?

4. Budget
    - How much would you budget for the program?

5. Strategy
    - What do you recommend to make the program successful?
    - What do you see as possible obstacles to be aware of and overcome?

6. Organization Priorities
    - What is the organization's mission?
    - What are the organization's long-term goals?
    - What are the organization's current priorities?

Middle managers are the final gatekeepers to the employees' participation in the program. The key question that must be answered about their support is: Will these managers allow, facilitate, and encourage their employees to participate in the programs?

Among the general employee population, the questions of support are simple ones: Do employees want the programs? Will they participate?

As simple as these questions are, measuring support is difficult because most people don't know what a health promotion program is and, worse yet, harbor false impressions. This was evidenced by one senior manager whose young wife was involved in competitive aerobics classes. He said he didn't want to do aerobics because he thought he would look silly wearing tights and dancing to music. He didn't realize aerobics includes a wide range of cardiovascular exercises (like running, swimming, and bicycling) and that none of these programs required wearing skimpy attire. Another middle manager did not want to take a stress management class because she equated this with meditation, which she felt was a form of faddish Eastern religion. She envisioned the group discussions as threatening encounter groups with sexual overtones. Another senior manager was afraid of health promotion programs because he thought he would have to build a fitness facility and talk people into becoming body builders. Another employee was nervous about participating in a health screening because she thought the results would be shared with her supervisor. Many employees have been concerned about participating in health screenings because they were concerned about losing medical insurance coverage.

Support must sometimes be measured indirectly because of these misconceptions. If a top manager wants to focus effort on reducing medical care costs and has a strong concern for her own well-being and the well-being of her employees, she can probably be counted as an advocate of the program because she supports what it stands for. An employee who wants to exercise more, stop smoking, eat better, or learn to relax and who also feels comfortable accepting guidance from her employer would probably be a supporter of the program even though she does not know what it is.

Personal interviews are probably the most accurate method to measure support in this context. The interview allows the analyst to assess the employees' understanding of the programs and factor that knowledge into the interpretation of their comments. The analyst also has the opportunity to explain the elements of a program and clear up any misconceptions. Unfortunately, interviews take a lot of time. They should be used with members of top management and key non-managers, but time usually will not permit extensive interviews with the general employee population.

Questionnaires are the most practical tool to use with large groups of employees, but they do have some limitations. One of the biggest limitations is that the analyst does not know how the employee's understanding of the questionnaire or misconceptions about health promotion programs might bias the answers. Validity and reliability testing can reduce this problem, but most health promotion managers do not know how to perform these tests. Also, response rates to such questionnaires are often less than 30% of the employee population. This is problematic because those who do not respond often have different opinions and practices than those that do respond. Group interviews, called focus groups, can supplement the information provided by questionnaires.

Questionnaires for managers might address the following issues:

- Perceptions of levels of specific problems in the organization in areas that may be impacted by the health promotion program
- Beliefs on the potential impact of a health promotion program in the organization's specific problem areas
- Managers' general level of support for the program
- Program content interests

Points to address in questionnaires sent to employees should cover the following:

- Current health practices in each health area (e.g., exercise, nutrition, etc.)
- Interest in improving health practices in each health area
- Interest in participating in programs sponsored by the employer in each health area
- Perception of how well the employer is encouraging positive health practices in each health area

Questionnaires to measure employee's health practices, interests, and levels of perceived organizational support can be developed internally or purchased from external vendors. External vendors can also take on the time-consuming task of tallying and summarizing responses. Developing a high-quality questionnaire is difficult and time consuming and should not be attempted unless the developer is skilled in this area. Newly developed questionnaires should be refined for clarity through pilot testing and analyzed for psychometric properties (validity and reliability) through further testing. Without this type of testing, it is not likely that the information collected by the questionnaire will be very useful. Also, it is critical that responses are received from a sufficiently large sample.

Vendors selling standardized questionnaires should be asked to demonstrate that their questionnaires have strong psychometric properties. Also, standardized questionnaires should be used only if they include the specific information relevant to the program design effort.

A growing number of vendors can develop custom questionnaires to address individual needs of different organizations, process the responses, and provide summary reports for a reasonable cost.

Some organizations use a **health risk assessment** (HRA) to collect information to design a program. This is a tempting strategy because the HRA does measure employee health risks and provide computer tallies of the results. This is now financially feasible because the cost of an online HRA is so low, however, because the HRA requires so much information from employees, the response rate is often low and biased toward people who are interested in making health improvements. As discussed later, response rates can be increased significantly with the appropriate promotion and incentives, but this is sometimes difficult to do during the planning process, i.e. before a program is fully launched.

Discussing specific questionnaire content is beyond the scope of this workbook. However, any questionnaire attempting to measure employee health behaviors and interest in participating in programs will be of limited value if it does not measure the employees readiness to change each health behavior.[5] Understanding stage of readiness to change is critical to preparing the types of programs most appropriate for the population and for projecting participation rates.

Access to Resources

The resources required to develop and operate the program include money, space, technical knowledge, and staff to run the programs. The organization's ability to finance the program is independent of the cost/benefit value of the program. In addition to recognizing the cost/benefit value, the organization must have access to liquid assets to develop and operate the program. An organization might project it will earn $2 for every $1 it invests in the program; but if it does not have sufficient cash reserves, it may not be able to start the program.

Space is often a problem for organizations located in or close to urban areas, especially when they want to provide fitness facilities. Fortunately, many programs do not require fitness facilities or extensive space.

Technical knowledge on program design, curriculum development, and health assessment—among other areas—is necessary to develop the program. Skilled staff are required to operate it. The organization must have these resources within its employee group or be able to contract for them in the community. Contracting for these services will not be a problem for most organizations in urban settings in the United States but may be difficult for organizations in small towns or in countries that do not have extensive health promotion capabilities.

Program Development Issues

After the organizational goals are clarified, the cost/benefit analysis is completed, levels of interest are measured, and support and access to resources are determined, the organization should be able to determine if it is feasible to develop a health promotion program. If it determines that the program is feasible, it should then address program development issues. The basic program development question it must answer is: If the health promotion program seems to be a good investment of the organization's resources and the organization can draw all the necessary resources from itself and the community, how should it proceed in developing the program? More specifically:

- What departments and individuals should be involved in developing the program?
- What are the various combinations of community and organizational resources that can be used to develop the program?
- Which of the program focus options seem to be most appropriate for achieving the stated organization and health goals?
- What will be the major obstacles to overcome in developing the program?

The answers to these questions give management a clear view of what is required to move to the next step—developing program content.

PHASE III: PROGRAM DESIGN – DEVELOPING PROGRAM CONTENT AND MANAGEMENT STRUCTURE

Program design is the third major phase in developing the program. Although this phase is described as having finite limits—starting after the feasibility study and ending before implementation—the actual design of the program will continue to evolve as it becomes integrated into the organization. This evolution will be visible if the program has a scheduled evaluation and readjustment phase or is implemented on a pilot or phased-in basis. The program will continue to evolve in all cases, even when the evolution is not visible.

Results of the Program Design Phase

Just as the feasibility study produces a guide to lead into the program design phase, the program design phase produces a plan for implementation. The plan should be directed by a clear statement of the health change or lifestyle goals and the organizational goals of the program. Specific descriptions of program contents, program and corporate-level management systems, financing arrangements, use of outside vendors, participant policies, and an implementation schedule should be included. In many cases, specific program curricula will be developed during the design phase. This will often be true less if the program is going or phased in slowly or if course curricula are to be supplied by an outside vendor.

Factors Influencing Program Design

The importance of clearly stating the program's organizational and health improvement goals in such a way that they can guide the design process has been discussed. Unfortunately, it is often very difficult to position the program's goals as the primary factor impacting the design of the program. Myriad political forces can often skew the focus of the design. A good program designer may be able to recognize these forces and channel them to support, rather than derail, the stated goals of the program in many cases. In other cases, the program designer may be able to recognize but not influence these factors.

Quality of the Design Process

The first challenge will be to ratify stated program goals that reflect the needs of the organization. Top management may have priorities different from managers and employees. The design team's lack of understanding of health promotion programs may further confuse the goal ratification process. The impact of these difficulties can be reduced by educating the design team on the history, operation, and expected benefits of health promotion programs.

Securing Employee Support

The problem of securing employee and middle-management support for programs proposed by top management is common for many programs in most large organizations. Extensive management processes have been developed to address this problem. The impact of the problem can be reduced if it receives appropriate attention. This is especially important in the design and implementation of a health promotion program because it affects each participant in a very personal way. The most effective strategy is probably to involve employees and managers in all aspects of the design and management of the program, to design the program to meet their specific needs, to keep them well-informed of program developments and make transparency a centerpiece of the program.

Impact of the Program on Design Committee Members' Jobs

The development of a program can have a major impact on the jobs of managers operationally linked to the program, e.g., benefits managers, facilities managers, training directors, and managers of employee health. The new program may increase their power base, threaten their turf, increase their workload, or expose the quality of their work. In fact, in most cases, a new health promotion program will focus new attention on the management of medical care costs, rates of absenteeism and turnover, and productivity levels. This is one of the spin-off benefits of the health promotion program. The program often provides a non-threatening environment in which to address these problems. Nevertheless, the initial exposure of these problems is often very threatening to the manager(s) in charge of these areas.

Knowledge and Experience of Design Committee Members

The background of the design team members will have a major impact on their input into the design process. A facilities manager may have an orientation toward fitness facilities, a training director toward classes, a nurse or physician toward screening programs, and a recreation leader toward sports and other fun events. Any exposure team members have had to other programs will further influence their input. If the same group were on a team designing a computer system, their biases would have less impact on their input because they would not feel knowledgeable about computers and would defer to those with technical expertise. However, most people feel they know a lot about health and health habits and can personalize the program to their own situation. Consequently they are more vocal and allow their own personal preferences to affect their input.

Profitability and Organization Transitions

Unrelated cycles of the organization will make a difference in the design of the program. These cycles can postpone the development of the program, speed up the process, or shift its focus. For example, a pending corporate relocation might postpone the program's development until the move is made. However, the construction of *new* corporate facilities and the initiation of new management programs that usually accompany such a move might facilitate implementation of the program. A high-profit year can free funds to develop the program. A low-profit year can make funds difficult to come by. Ironically, an organization in a poor profit situation especially needs to enhance productivity, reduce medical care costs, and correct image problems that health promotion programs address. Further, the cost of a health promotion program is usually not so great that it would be a significant drain on funds. Nevertheless, in tight financial times, new programs and programs not contributing directly to the core business of the organization are often discontinued or delayed.

DESIGN OPTIONS: PROGRAM CONTENTS

Design decisions made during the design phase focus on the contents of the program, the organizational system to manage the program, and the policies governing participation in the program.

The three major decisions made about program contents center on (a) the desired level of impact of the program, (b) the desired intensity of the program, and (c) the topics covered by the program.

Level of Impact

The most important decision on program content is the level of impact desired. As discussed earlier, programs that focus on enhancing *awareness* have the impact of increasing knowledge but have very little impact on behavior. *Skill building* programs help people change specific health behaviors, such as quitting smoking, starting to exercise, learning to manage stress, etc. Unfortunately, after people complete these programs, they often revert to their previous unhealthy lifestyles.[6] People will be much more likely to continue to practice healthy lifestyles on a long-term basis when they have *opportunities* that make the healthy choice the easiest choice.

Supportive cultural environments were one of the eight characteristics of the most successful programs discovered in the benchmarking study. The most successful programs take a comprehensive approach.[7] Also, as shown in Table 4, it is important to stress that programs with all four elements of the AMSO framework are ones most likely to achieve the organizational goals that most employers want to achieve.

Level of Intensity

The level of intensity of the program is determined by the degree of success desired in the health change goal and the level of intensity needed to achieve success. For example, in smoking cessation, systematic reviews of the literature have shown that quit rates increase as the number of minutes of counseling increase to 300, as the number of sessions increase to eight, the number of professionals leading the program reaches three, and a combination of behavior therapy and medication are used.[8] A supportive environment that includes extensive exercise facilities, frequent incentives to practice healthy behavior, and top management support will have a greater chance of success than a less intensive program. Factors determining the level of intensity include the quantity of resources invested, staff levels provided, and time spent by the participants in the programs. The increased intensity of the program will translate to increased success to the extent that the program is well designed. The most appropriate level of intensity will also be determined by the health conditions and health practices of specific employees. Given that a small portion of the employees are responsible for a majority of the medical care costs, it will be advisable to provide high-intensity programs to these employees if the goal of the program is to reduce medical care costs or to reach those with the greatest health risks.

Program Topics

Selection of topics will be relatively easy once the program goals are clearly stated and the desired level and intensity of the program are determined. Table 9 shows the type of programs that might be most appropriate for different health goals. Table 10 shows the type of programs that might be most appropriate for different organization goals. Both of these tables of programs were developed by a health promotion design committee designing an actual program. They are not intended to be the only programs appropriate for the health and organization problem areas shown. In many cases the program's health goals are not very specific and are instead directed toward improving employees' overall well-being. In those cases, a broad range of topics is normally advisable, and program topics might be selected based on what is expected to be most popular.

Table 9

Programs Most Appropriate for Health Goals

Hypertension	**Obesity**
Medical evaluation and prescription	Fitness
Nutrition & fitness	Nutrition
Weight control	Self-esteem training
Smoking cessation	Stress management
Stress management	Weight control
Stress	**Smoking**
Fitness	Smoking policy
Childcare	Smoking cessation
Employee assistance program (EAP)	Fitness
Policy review	Weight control
Stress management	Stress management

Table 10

Programs Most Appropriate for Organization Goals

High Medical Care Costs	Low Morale	Low Productivity
Medical self-care	Dependent care	Policy review
Risk rating	facilities & programs	Fitness programs
Hypertension control	Visible fitness facilities	Dependent care
Injury control	Employee Assistance	facilities & programs
Smoking policy	Programs (EAPs)	Stress management
Smoking cessation	Policy review	Comprehensive
Medical coverage	Incentive programs	programs
	Recreation programs	
	Other visible programs	

Also, it is valuable to be able to offer programs that are appropriate to each of the major stages of readiness to change for each of the health behavior areas. For example, the needs assessment might show that 25% of the employees are smokers, and that 40% of smokers are in the precontemplation stage, 40% are in the contemplation, and 20% are in preparation. Only the employees in preparation will likely be ready to quit and would want to participate in a formal quit-smoking program. In an organization with 1,000 employees, these values would translate to 250 smokers, 50 of whom are ready to quit. If half of them were able to sign up for a quit-smoking course right away, that would translate to 25 smokers. A classic face-to-face quit program focusing on quitting smoking would thus be helpful to only 10% of all the smokers. A core advantage of most web-based and telephone coaching approaches is that they are designed to serve the needs of employees at all of the stages of readiness to change. An additional advantage is that there are no minimum numbers of employees that can participate at one time, and maximums can usually be handled if some warning is given...although there are some limits to the number of telephone coaches that can be available at any one time on short notice. Table 11 shows strategies that might be appropriate for each of the stages of readiness to change. These strategies can be adapted to each of the health behavior areas.

Table 11

Strategies Based on Motivational Readiness to Change

Precontemplation
- Unconditional acceptance
- Indirect comments

Contemplation
- Enhance behavioral efficacy
- Enhance self efficacy
- Expose social networks
- Aspirational goal setting

Preparation
- Learning goal setting
- Enhance self efficacy
- Enhance behavioral efficacy
- Introduce to social networks

Action
- Performance goal setting
- Skill building
- Engage in social networks

Maintenance
- Maintain social networks
- Offer leadership opportunities
- Reinforce self efficacy
- Reinforce behavioral efficacy

Communication, Incentives and Supportive Cultures

The final three components of the best programs in benchmarking are effective communication efforts, incentive efforts, and supportive cultures.

Effective communication programs serve the basic purpose of enhancing employee awareness about the links between health behaviors and health outcomes, but equally important, they make employees aware of many program offerings available to help them improve health practices. The most effective communication efforts are tailored to the individual characteristics of employees, including their personal priorities in life, and their motivational readiness to change. The best communication programs need to be ubiquitous to reach a large portion of the employee population, and meet high quality standards to convey a high quality health promotion program.

The primary impact of incentive programs is to enhance participation. This is critically important because only the employees in preparation will be ready to join actual programs, and this typically represents a small portion of the population, perhaps as low as 20% of employees. Incentives may be an effective way to attract the attention of the other 80% of the employees. Incentives can be intrinsic, focusing on internal values, or extrinsic, focusing on cash awards and prices. They can take the form of simple, small-prize giveaways to people who attend an event, cash to people who complete a health screening, chances in lotteries for larger prizes, discounts on health plan premiums, or other forms. Well designed incentive programs have been shown to push participation rates to the 70% to 90% range,[9,10] however, there is little evidence that incentive programs have much impact in actually changing health behaviors.[11]

People's health behaviors are strongly influenced by the behavioral norms of their friends, family, co-workers and society at large. It is more difficult to eat junk food, take the elevator and smoke when everyone around you is eating nutritious food, taking the stairs and never smoking. Organizations with the best health promotion programs have been able to create organization cultures that facilitate positive health practices and have programs consistent with behavior change theories.

DEVELOPING A MANAGEMENT STRUCTURE

Important management decisions to be made during the design process include where to place the program in the organizational structure, how much staffing is required, how to build strong top management support, how to finance the program, how often to use vendors and consultants, who will be eligible to participate, what will be the necessary operating procedures, and how to evaluate the program. Each of these issues is discussed briefly below.

Location in the Organizational Structure

The placement of the health promotion program in the organization will depend on the focus of the program and the related organizational goals; rank within the organizational hierarchy; and personalities, images, and workloads of various departments.

Program Focus and Goals

It makes sense to pair the program with the department most closely responsible for achieving the health or organizational goals the program is designed to achieve. If the program goal is educational, the training and development department might be most appropriate. A program centered on health screening and risk reduction might fit best in the medical or employee health department. A fitness facility with very little programming could be supervised by the facility's management department. The benefits department might be appropriate if the program is designed to reduce health care expenditures. A recreation-centered program might fit well within the employee association. If the program focus is broader and is designed to improve the overall well-being of the employees, direct management by the human resources department probably makes the most sense.

Organizational Hierarchy

The health promotion program should be at a level high enough in the organization that the manager has direct access to top management when necessary and is on the same level as line managers supervising the employees who will be enrolled in the programs.

Personalities, Images, Work Loads of Managers and Department

A new health promotion program is in a precarious position. Because it is a new concept that is sometimes not very well-understood, much of its long-term success will depend on how well it is positioned at its inception. Ideally, the department responsible for the health promotion program should have a positive image. The manager supervising the program director should be well-respected, very supportive of the concept, a good role model, and have sufficient time to give strong support for the program during its inception.

Linkages with Other Departments

The health promotion program will normally be designed to achieve numerous organizational goals, including reducing health care expenditures, improving the corporate image, reducing absenteeism, and increasing work output. In most cases, specific departments in the organization are responsible for each of these areas. Therefore, each of these departments should be linked to the health promotion program. Additionally, other departments—such as communications, public relations, and plant management–will be important to the successful day-to-day operation of the program and should also be linked to the program. Finally, the participation of the employees from all departments in the organization is critical to the growth and survival of the program. Linkages to all of these staff support departments and to line managers in other departments should therefore be established.

The optimal mechanism for the linkage to each of these groups will be different in each case. Committees are appropriate in some cases; however, in order to be effective, they should have clear tasks and be well-managed. Recruiting key managers and employees to serve as volunteers in responsible operational roles in the program can also work.

If the program is managed by a support department such as human resources, additional links should be made directly to top management. One method is to appoint a top line manager as a figurehead leader of the program. The program manager would be responsible for all administrative functions, but the figurehead top manager would be available for troubleshooting and public relations efforts. This is analogous to the city manager / mayor form of government used in some cities or the executive director/ honorary national chairperson of a national campaign.

Staffing Levels

The benchmarking study determined that the best programs have approximately one full-time professional staff person for every 1800 employees. This figure is also consistent with the staffing ratio recommended by a number of major program management companies.

Modeling Best Programs to Build Top Management Support

Having strong top management support is one of the characteristics of the best health promotion programs. Which came first? In most cases, the former *preceded* the latter. Many programs become excellent because they have strong top management support. Regardless of the current level of top management support, program developers should focus on this point as they develop their program. First, they should tell top management that strong support is one of the eight ingredients for a successful program. This may motivate some top managers to become more involved. Second, developers should ask top managers what they need to do to insure strong support from top management, make sure those things are done, and make sure top management knows these things are being done. As discussed earlier, one of the most important factors in developing top management support is linking the program to the organization's goals and making top management aware of how the program is supporting those goals.

Program Budgets and Funding
Budgets

There are no standardized recommendations on how much to budget for a comprehensive health promotion program. However, examining the budgets of successful programs can provide some guidance.

A meta analysis of 22 programs that had **returns on investment (ROI)** of 3.27 in medical cost savings and 22 programs that had returns on investment of 2.73 in absenteeism reduction reported annual budgets that averaged $144 per person and $132 per person (2009 dollars) respectively. Despite their success in producing impressive savings, their level of comprehensiveness is not known.[12]

The benchmarking study found that the average annual budget among the best programs was approximately $200 per eligible employee (not per participant) in 1996 dollars. This is consistent with the author's experience that an internally managed comprehensive program that includes awareness, motivation, skill building and opportunities costs approximately $205 (in 2012 dollars) per employee (not per participant) in an organization with at least 4,000 employees. These figures include staff salaries but do not include office space, employee benefits, overhead benefits, staff recruitment, initial training costs, or the cost of top management's supervision of the program. If fitness facilities are included, this will add an additional $100 to $200 per employee (not per participant), including amortization of construction costs over 15 years but not including land acquisition or space costs. Fitness facility costs can often be reduced by charging employees a modest membership fee.

Despite the significant expansion of the scope of the typical program in the past decade, the cost of the typical comprehensive program has not increased substantially in that period. Cost increases have been moderated in part by the cost effectiveness of web based HRAs and skill-building programs, which can often be provided for 10% to 20% of the cost of paper and pencil HRAs and in-person skill building programs. The rate of increase has also been much lower than the annual increase in medical care costs. As a result, the ability of programs to break even and to produce substantial returns on investment in medical cost savings has improved over the last decade.

Program Funding

Employers fund health promotion programs through four basic approaches, and often supplement this funding with a variety of these sources. These are listed and described below.

1. Perfunctory budgeting strategies.
2. Projected medical cost savings and productivity enhancements.

3. Integration into health plan premium.
4. Not hiring smokers.
5. Health plan supplements, vendor guarantees, employee fees.

Perfunctory Budgeting Strategies

Most employers, especially small- and medium-sized employers, fund their health promotion ef-forts the same way they fund every other relatively small operational purchase they make. Cost of health promotion programs are similar to the costs of office supplies, office furniture, landscaping, office parties, sports leagues, interior decorating. Given a cost of $250 per employee per year for a comprehensive program, employers realize that health promotion programs are a cost ef-fective way to help employees improve their health, and to attract and retain the most talented workforce. The cost is half the cost of a 1% raise for a person who makes $50,000 a year and 4% of the $6000/covered life they spend for employee health insurance each year. Employers who purchase health promotion programs with this mindset, focus on getting the best price for the program that meets their needs, and typically monitor employee participation and satisfac-tion, but do not attempt to measure medical cost savings or productivity enhancements. This approach is most common among small to medium sized employers who self fund their health plans.

Projected Medical Cost Savings and Productivity Enhancements

Most large employers think of their health promotion programs as investments that are likely to reduce medical costs and absenteeism, help attract and retain the best employees, and possibly enhance productivity. They are under extreme pressure to control the rate of increase in their medical care costs, and are often familiar with the literature which shows that more than 60 well-designed programs have reduced medical costs and absenteeism[13] and nearly two dozen programs have seen medical care cost savings of approximately $3 for every dollar invested plus absenteeism cost savings nearly as high, producing a total ROI of 6:1.[14] They also know that savings are not likely in the first year, breakeven is possible in the second year, and net savings are likely to be realized by the third year of the program. They might not expect to see savings of this order of magnitude from their own programs, and they usually realize that few if any product lines in their own organization produce ROIs of 6:1, but they do believe it is very likely their invest-ment in health promotion will save more than it costs in hard dollars. They are also aware that a well-designed program can enhance employee well-being and morale. These employers work hard to get the best possible price from the vendors they hire and usually focus programs in areas that will produce financial returns. Most of them are not prepared to spend the several hundred thousand dollars necessary to conduct a well designed study on the financial return of their programs, but they do want to closely monitor effective implementation of program components, expect high levels of employee participation and satisfaction, and focus on changes in employee health risks and health conditions. They are interested in their vendors' estimates of cost savings, but may not take them too seriously.

Integrate into Health Plan

The author predicts an emerging trend, especially among large self-insured employers, in which the full cost of the health promotion program will be included in the organization's medical plan costs. The $250/person/year typical annual cost of a comprehensive health promotion program represents only 4% of the typical $6000/employee/year cost of a typical health plan. This puts the low cost of the health promotion program, relative to health plan costs, into sharp focus. The employer, then, has the option of passing some, or all, of the program cost to employees in the form of slightly higher premium payments. For example, if the employer covered 70% of the health plan cost and employees covered the 30% balance, and the same formula was applied to the health promotion program, the employee would cover $83.33 (30% x $250) of the cost, or $7/month. If the program is successful in reducing medical costs as expected, the cost increase should pay for itself in the second year and produce savings in excess of costs by the third year, resulting in no net cost to the employee or employer.

An important enabler of this emerging trend is the integration of health promotion financial incentives into medical plan premiums among large self-insured employers. Through these incentives, the amount of an employee's health plan premium is in part tied to their success in achieving health goals or participating in programs to achieve those goals. The net result is that employees who achieve all of their health goals or choose to participate in programs to achieve those goals, pay the lowest premiums, and employees who choose not to participate pay the highest premiums. A survey of large employers showed that 36% offered financial incentives for participating in programs and 8% for achieving health goals in 2009 and this grew to 80% for participation and 38% for health outcomes in 2012.[15] The major stimulus of this growth is Section 2705 of the Affordable Care Act (ACA), which confirmed in statute what was previously only in federal regulation, that employers can provide a discount on the total health plan cost for employees who participate in programs or meet health standards. The ACA confirmed the discount to be 20% through the end of 2013, specified that it would increase to at least 30% in 2014 and allowed the Secretaries of Health and Human Services and Treasury to increase the differential to as high as 50% in 2014. Regulations guiding the implementation of section 2705 were released on behalf of the Departments of Treasury, Health and Human Services, and Labor May 29, 2013, and published in the Federal Register on June 3, 2013, just a few weeks before this text went into production.[16] As such, employers and consultants are still sorting through the exact meaning of the 36 dense pages of legalese and are trying to translate what is allowed and prohibited into incentive program design. A further complication is that the agencies expect to release additional "subregulations" based on questions posed by the public or misinterpretations caused by incomplete detail in these regulations. In addition, the Equal Employment Opportunity Commission (EEOC) has not yet released its regulations. Some employers are delaying implementation of new incentive programs until the dust settles on these issues, while others are moving forward. Appendix A provides a description of an approach to integrate financial incentives for health promotion programs into health plan premiums that is consistent with the regulations, cost neutral to employers, and likely to motivate the vast majority of employees to get involved in the health promotion program. This approach is likely to be refined in the coming months and years. This approach is grounded in empirical literature related to program participation and equity.

Program Participation. Two separate studies showed that health promotion programs with well-designed marketing efforts and strong support from top management had participation rates in the 20% to 40% range, while those that also offered financial incentives to participate had rates in the 70% to 90% range;[17] those in the 90% range integrated their incentives into the health plan design.[18] Using this approach to providing incentives could lead to near universal participation in health promotion programs among employees who work in organizations that offer this approach, and thus significant improvements in the health of these employees.

Health Plan Cost Equity. A study of 46,026 employees in six different organizations found that employees with no health risk factors had medical costs 70% lower than those with multiple risk factors.[19] This means that employees who are working hard to successfully manage their health but are required to pay the same premium as other employees, are being forced to subsidize employees who are not even willing to participate in programs to improve their help. Offering a 20%, 30%, or 50% premium discount to employees who achieve health goals or participate in programs to try to improve, reduces the inequity, but also continues to provide a more than fair arrangement for those who choose not to participate.

Not Hire Smokers

The American Civil Liberties Union estimated that at least 6,000 employers had policies of not hiring smokers.[20] Some, including hospitals and voluntary health organizations, adopted these policies to be consistent with their health missions. Some employers take this approach to reduce exposure of employees and customers to second hand smoke and to encourage their employees to quit. Second hand smoke alone kills an estimated 53,000, more than are killed by car crashes.[21] Smoking remains the top preventable cause of death in the United States, killing more than 400,000 people each year. This is more each year than all the deaths of all Americans in all of the foreign wars in our history.[22] Most smokers (79.3%) expect to quit at some point, a majority (58.4%) plan to do so within the next 6 months, and many of them (46.8%) actually try to quit each year,[23] so many smokers who already have jobs in these companies welcome such a policy because it gives them an extra nudge to quit. Other employers, including manufacturers who deal with toxic explosive chemicals adopt these policies for safety reasons. Finally, some employers don't hire smokers to save money. The Centers for Disease Control and Prevention estimated the annual direct medical costs of smoking at $1,623 in 1998 dollars, and the indirect costs, including time off work for smoking breaks, at $1,760 [24] for a total of $3,383 per year per smoker. Not hiring smokers provides an immediate payoff to any employer who hires new employees on a regular basis. For example, an employer with 1,000 employees, annual turnover rate of 15%, a smoking rate of 20% among new hires, and an average annual cost of $3,000 per smoker (reduced from the $3,383 estimate of CDC) who implemented a policy of not hiring smokers would save $90,000 in the first year, an additional $166,500 in the second year, and an additional $231,525 in the third year. The policy would save a total of $3,269,373 by the 10th year, $769,373 more than had been spent on the comprehensive employee health promotion during that decade. This is in addition to medical cost savings produced by the health promotion program, which would be expected to be in the $7 million range for the decade.[25]

Employers who adopt these policies report that they have few negative repercussions, among existing employees or in their communities, especially when they assure existing employees who smoke that they will not be forced to quit smoking and that their smoking status will not impact job security. However, some employers choose not to implement these policies because they are concerned about employee or community backlash.

Furthermore, not hiring smokers might not be advisable for organizations with labor shortages, especially if they need to hire large numbers of blue-collar workers, or other workers with high smoking rates. Also, employers should be aware of laws governing hiring in their states. Twenty-one states (Alabama, Alaska, Arizona, Arkansas, Delaware, Florida, Georgia, Hawaii, Idaho, Iowa, Kansas, Maryland, Massachusetts, Michigan, Nebraska, Ohio, Pennsylvania, Texas, Utah, Vermont, Washington), have no restrictions on not hiring smokers. The remaining 29 states and the District of Columbia have passed laws elevating smokers to protected status. Not hiring smokers in those states is prohibited unless the reason is job related.[26]

Health Plan Funding, Employee Fees and Vendor Guarantees

Health plan funding. Some employers are able to supplement program funding with contributions from health plans and employee fees and secure guarantees of saving or reimbursement of costs from vendors. For example, a survey of a national representative sample of 730 employers reported that 47.7% of employers that had health promotion programs listed their health plan as the primary funder of their health promotion program.[27] Similarly, in a more recent survey of 1,515 firms, 87% of all firms reported that most of their wellness benefits are provided by their health plan.[28] The portion was 88% for firms with 3-199 employees, 68% for firms with 200 or more employees and 56% for firms with 5,000 or more employees The programs offered by health plans at no cost are typically online portals that can include health risk assessment screenings; skill building programs on fitness, nutrition, stress management, weight control, smoking cessation and medical self-care; and online chat groups. These programs can provide a valuable supplement to the program elements provided by the employers, but do not, by themselves, provide all the components necessary for a comprehensive programs.

Employee fees. Employers tend to avoid charging employee fees for most components of their health promotion program because they want to remove all barriers to entry. In fact, they often give employees financial incentives to join the programs. However, it is not unusual to charge fees for membership to onsite health clubs or for programs that provide nutritious meals.

Vendor guarantees. An emerging trend that may or may not last, is for vendors to guarantee medical care cost savings that exceed program costs in exchange for sharing a portion of those savings with the vendor. Employers are normally required to follow specific implementation protocols to qualify for the guarantee. This is an interesting approach that could motivate late adopting employers to implement programs, however, there is minimal documentation on the success of this approach. One of the unintended consequences of this approach might be that employers would have an incentive to show that programs have not saved money while vendors would have an incentive to show they do save money. This could lead to conflicts between employers and providers, and different interpretations of the same data. Vendor guarantees are described in more details in Appendix C.

Given the range of funding options available to employers, and the high likelihood of a positive financial return, the financial barriers to implementing a health program might be described as minimal, a least for moderate to large employers.

Use of Vendors and Consultants

In the United States, vendors and consultants are available to serve virtually all the employer's needs related to the health promotion program. They can design the program, hire staff, build facilities, manage programs, conduct health screenings, provide face-to-face and online skill-building programs, supply materials and equipment, and evaluate programs. They can do this on a turnkey basis or piece-by-piece.

The criteria and methods used to determine whether to use vendors, how much to use them, and how to select them should be the same as those used in evaluating the use of vendors for other projects. The employer's experience in going through the same questions in developing the organization's health insurance plan, its computer capabilities, or its facilities can be helpful. The individual responsible for these decisions should have some knowledge of health promotion and be skilled in dealing with vendors. However, health promotion programs are different from computer systems in that they impact employees in a very personal way. If outside vendors are used to provide programs, effective integration of the human factor needs to be a top criteria in vendor selection. Employees need to feel that they, and not the vendor, own the program.

When all the hidden costs of an internally managed program are considered, the costs of managing a program internally and externally are comparable. Working with an outside vendor also has the additional advantages of being able to get a program started quickly without hiring new staff, and being able to terminate it when the contract period has passed, without needing to layoff any staff. It is not surprising that a large portion of workplace health promotion programs are now managed by external vendors.

Eligibility for the Program

The magnitude of the program and the method of deciding who is eligible to participate in the program should be determined during the design phase. The program can be made available to all employees or only to selected employees. The program can also be offered to spouses, children, unmarried partners, and retirees. The eligibility policy should be determined by the goals for the program and the resources available to develop it. The program might start as a small pilot project and grow on a phased-in basis until it becomes available to all employees and family. In other cases, it might start small and stay small. It might be offered to employees in one division or location; to top management; to employees with specific health conditions; to a random cross section of all employees; or on a first-come, first-served basis.

Family participation is important if a core program goal is improving health habits because it is very difficult for an employee to change a health habit without the support of close family members. This is especially true for tobacco use and nutrition. Similarly, involving the family is important if the goal is to reduce medical care costs because spouses and dependents might account for up to three-quarters of all medical claims. Given the growing pressure for most employers to reduce their medical costs, the general trend over the past decade has been for employers to engage as many employees in programs as fast as possible, and to be less concerned about the marginal program costs for each additional employee. Employers have begun to work to engage spouses and children, but most have had only limited success.

Operating Procedures

Procedures for operating the program should be outlined during the design phase. These procedures will include staffing plans, scheduling, promotional methods, facilities maintenance, budgeting, materials and equipment management, and evaluation methods. Some of the details of these procedures will be refined during implementation and initial operation.

Evaluation Plan

An evaluation effort is an important part of every health promotion program. The benchmarking study showed that the best programs have evaluation efforts in place, and equally important, that they communicate their evaluation results. In addition to measuring the impact of the program on health outcomes, the evaluation effort should measure the extent to which it addresses the organization's long-term goals and current priorities. Of course, these findings should be communicated to top management.

The evaluation plan—including what will be evaluated, when it will be evaluated, how, by whom and for what purpose—should be specified as the program plan is developed. If the evaluation plan is not developed and approved as part of the basic program plan, it will be very difficult to start the evaluation once the program is up and running. Also, some baseline measures will need to be recorded before programs are launched so that progress against these values can be assessed. If the evaluation plan is not developed, it will be difficult to know which baseline measures need to be taken.

Approximately 5 to 10% of the program budget should be allocated to program evaluation to effectively monitor the implementation of the program and its effectiveness.

Modeling other Successful Programs

A useful exercise for advanced program developers is to review what has been written about the most highly recognized programs. The Health Project has assembled descriptions of programs that have been awarded the prestigious C. Everett Koop Award based on the success of these programs in improving health, reducing medical costs and enhancing productivity. These are featured on their website.[29]

Scorecards developed by the Health Enhancement Research Organization (HERO) and the Centers for Disease Control and Prevention (CDC) provide an excellent reference for planning a program. These scorecards were developed primarily to audit and guide the refinement of existing programs, but they can also be used proactively to serve as a road map for the development of new programs. They are briefly described in Appendix D.

CONCLUSION

One of the biggest challenges facing all health promotion professionals is adapting their content training in exercise, education, psychology, nutrition, nursing, or any other clinical area to work settings. Very few of these professionals receive training in management procedures. This becomes very evident when they attempt to design a workplace health promotion program. Fortunately, protocols like those described here have been developed that work. Our challenge in health promotion program design is not so much to develop better design techniques but to make health promotion professionals aware that they exist and to improve their ability to follow them.

The next challenge for employers will be to reach beyond the workplace, into the schools, faith communities, and the other organizations in which people spend their time when they are not at work, and in which spouses and children spend their time. These efforts might even include collaborating with the employers of spouses. The goal of these outreach efforts would be to weave a web of support that reaches people several times each day with the most effective strategies where they work, shop, study, worship and relax.

Appendix A

**Integrating Financial Incentives into Health Plan Design based on Section 2705
of the Affordable Care Act and Subsequent Regulations**

Background

Section 2705 of the Affordable Care Act confirmed that group health plans, including self-insured employers, may adjust health plan premiums based on employees participating in health promotion programs and achieving health goals. Final regulations describing how this law could be applied were published in the Federal Register on June 3, 2013. The recommendations on how to integrate these new regulations into health plan premium design are described below, with three cautions. 1) These recommendations were written just 10 days after the regulations were released and will no doubt be refined as the intention of specific sections of the regulations become more clear. 2) The agencies expect to release subregulations based on questions from the public and misinterpretations of the regulations. 3) The Equal Employment Opportunity Commission has not yet released its regulations.

Key Provisions of the Federal Regulations

The federal regulations are presented in a format and tone that no doubt make sense to lawyers and regulators, but are baffling to the typical health promotion professional. The key elements of the federal regulations are summarized below in greatly abbreviated form, and in terms that are more likely to be understandable to health promotion professionals

Intention of the Federal Regulations

Language in the federal regulations makes it clear that the authors of the regulations want to make it possible for employees who chose to participate in health promotion programs to receive the full discount, even if they do not achieve specified health goals. On page 33160, they state the following: "The intention of the Departments in these final regulations is that, regardless of the type of wellness program, every individual participating in the program should be able to receive the full amount of any reward or incentive, regardless of any health factor." They operationalize this intention through the concept of an "alternative standard," which essentially allows anyone who does not meet any health goal an alternative method (or alternative standard to meet) to earn the discount. However, later language makes is clear that the authors are not attempting to eviscerate discounts based on achieving health outcomes. On page 33165 they state the following: "The requirement to provide a reasonable alternative standard to all individuals who do not meet or achieve a particular health outcome is not intended to transform all outcome-based wellness programs to participatory wellness programs." These two intentions in the regulations, which initially seem contradictory, should guide the design of any incentive program integrated into health plan premium structure.

Types of Incentive Structures

The federal regulations recognize three basic types of incentive structures (although they refer to these types of incentive programs as types of "wellness programs" instead of incentive structures). 1) *Participatory.* The most basic incentive program is based on a reward or discount being provided based on an employee merely participating in a program, such as a health screening, a lecture series, etc., without any requirement to meet a health goal. 2) *Activity-Only.* The next level of incentive program is based on a reward or discount being provided based on an employee completing an activity such as a running program, following a specific diet, etc. 3) *Outcome-Based.* The final level of incentive program is based on achieving a specific health goal, such as not using tobacco, having normal biometric values, normal weight, passing a fitness test, etc.

The only restrictions on *Participatory* incentives are to make them available to all "similarly situated individuals" (i.e. employees covered by the health plan, and their covered dependents if the health promotion program and incentive program is extended to them). *Activity-Only* and *Outcome-Based* incentive programs must meet five criteria: 1) allow people the opportunity to qualify at least once a year, 2) limit rewards to 30% of the total health plan premium, or 50% if tobacco use is part of the incentive, 3) be offered in the context of a health promotion program with a "reasonable design" that is likely to help the employee improve their health, 4) provide an "alternative standard" that an employee can meet if they are not able to perform the original activity or achieve the health standard (the employer can require physician verification of a medical reason the employee cannot perform the activity, but cannot require this for not meeting the health goal), 5) the means to achieve the alternative standard must be included in all promotional documents that describe the details of how to earn the incentive. The reward limits and the alternative standard are described in more detail below.

Amount of Discounts

Through the end of 2013, the maximum reward or discount is 20% of the total value of the health plan premium, including the employer and employee contribution. Beginning in 2014, the maximum discount increases to 30%, with the provision that an extra 20% can be added to programs that target tobacco use, for a total of 50%. The full amount of the discount must be "paid" in the year in which it is earned, even if the employee meets the standard at the end of the year and after cycling through a series of alternative standards over the span of the year. If necessary, it can be "paid" retroactively. The discount can be limited to the premium for the employee or can include the premium for spouses and dependents if they have convenient access to all aspects of the program. Employers have discretion on how to allocate the reward based on the "performance" of the individual family members in meeting or not meeting the various standards. Besides the requirement to include tobacco use in rewards of 50% versus 30%, there are no limitations on how the 30% reward can be allocated to various elements of the incentive program.

Alternative Standard

An alternative standard to earn the reward must be offered to all employees who are not able to meet the initial standard for *Activity-Only* or *Outcome-Based* incentives (but not for *Participatory* incentives). The alternative standard can be in the form of another incentive program with the same or a different structure. For example, for an employee who cannot meet the *Outcome-Based* standard of BMI of 25, the alternative standard could be meeting a fitness standard (another outcome standard), making progress in reducing weight to achieve a BMI of 27 (another outcome standard), participating in a program to increase physical activity or eating more nutritious foods *(Activity-Only* standard), or listening to a series of lectures on weight management (a *Participatory* standard). The alternative standard must always be "reasonable" and the opinion of the employee's personal physician must always prevail in the selection of the alternative standard if there is a disagreement.

Recommended Incentive Structure

Guiding Principles. The recommended incentive structure described below is designed with the goal of complying with the provisions in the regulation, motivating employees to be engaged in efforts to improve health, making the full cost of the incentive cost neutral to the employer, and having a premium structure that covers a portion of the cost of the health promotion program. Actual reductions in employer medical care costs would need to come from reduced medical care utilization caused by improved health or wiser use of medical care by employees.

This approach is based on a series of parallel incentive programs with the alternative standard for each of them being a related effort that benefits the employee's health.

Behavior and Health Conditions Targeted. I recommend keeping the structure of the incentive program simple so employees understand it and data management is not too cumbersome. I recommend focusing on one behavior (a *Participatory* incentive) which is participating in a health screening, and three health standards (*Outcome-Based* incentives) that can be measured objectively. Those health standards might be (1) no tobacco use, (2) body mass index (BMI) ≤27.5 or passing a fitness test, and (3) biometrics in the normal range, including blood pressure, cholesterol, triglycerides, and glucose. Values for all of these standards would need to be measured through screenings, not self reported, to avoid creating an incentive for employees to lie in a self-report.

Health Screening. The health screening needs to be conducted at least once a year, and measure all the health values covered by the other elements of the incentive program, including cotinine or another objective measure of tobacco use. Receiving an incentive for participating in a health screening is a *Participatory* level incentive, so no alternative standard is required.

Tobacco Use. The standard to receive the tobacco use incentive should be no measureable cotinine detected in the health screening. This would apply to employees using nicotine replacement therapy to quit smoking. This is an *Outcome-Based* level incentive, which requires an alternative standard option. The alternative standard should be the opportunity to participate in a tobacco cessation program. Receiving an incentive to participate in the tobacco cessation program is a *Participatory* level incentive and requires no alternative standard for employees who decide not to participate.

Recommended Weight. The standard to receive the recommended weight standard should be BMI of 27.5, or when possible, a comparable level from the direct measurement of body fat through an objective standard, with the employee choosing the measurement approach. The 27.5 BMI is recommended rather than the usual 25 BMI to provide slack for those who are moderately overweight and to recognize the inconsistent findings on the links between overweight (but not obesity) and health. Use of body fat percentage is recommended to account for employees who are heavy because of extensive muscle rather than excess fat. The alternative standard for this *Outcome-Based* level incentive would be another *Outcome-Based* level incentive of passing a fitness test. Passing a fitness test as an alternative standard is recommended because compelling research has shown that lack of fitness is a more important predictor of mortality than being overweight.[30] The alternative standard for this *Outcome-Based* level incentive might include a range of options including making progress in loosing weight or improving fitness (another *Outcome-Based* level), participating in a program to improve fitness and lose weight (an *Activity-Only* level or *Participatory* program, depending on the focus of the program). The choice of *Outcome-Based*, *Activity-Only*, or *Participatory* level incentives should be guided by the resources and overall philosophy of the health promotion program staff. The number of levels of alternative standards to be met should be guided by what the field learns over time about how long program participants will embrace vs. reject these multiple levels, and the culture of the employer organization.

Biometric Values. The standard for biometric values incentive should be recommended normal values for blood pressure, cholesterol (including ratios), glucose or Hemoglobin A_1c, and possibly triglycerides. The alternative standard for this *Outcome-Based* level incentive should be complying with appropriate medical care from a physician (an *Activity-Only* level incentive). Following the advice of a personal physician is also the final default alternative standard specific in the federal regulations for any *Outcome-Based* incentive. Another option is to combine the requirement to comply with physician advice with participation in programs to improve nutrition, fitness, manage stress, or lose weight.

Amounts of Incentives. The regulations allow considerable leeway in the amount of the incentive applied to individual components. A maximum incentive of 50% of the health plan premium is more than enough to capture an employee's attention and motivate them to become engaged in programs. Assuming average total medical care premium costs of $6000/person, 50% would be $3000... an amount that is probably more than enough to engage most employees. In earlier recommendations, when I assumed that maximum incentives levels would be 20% or 30%, I recommended incentives of 5% - 7.5% for participating in the screening, and 5% - 7.5% for achieving each of the three health goals.[31] This was based in part on my personal experience that $300 is probably enough to motivate most employees to participate in each distinct program, like participating in a health screening, or a tobacco cessation program. Given the new limit of 50%, I am inclined to increase the ranges, but am not able to justify these amounts with a cohesive rationale for increasing them at this point. Below are the ranges I think should be considered.

Participating in a health screening:	5% - 15%
No tobacco use:	5% - 20%
Meeting weight standard:	5% - 10%
Meeting biometric standard:	5% - 10%

I look forward to revising these ranges based employers' practical experience and the findings of scientists.

Appendix B

Proposed Regulations to Guide Implementation of Wellness Incentives in the Affordable Care Act

On November 20, 2012, proposed regulations to guide the implementation of the Wellness Incentives (Section 2705 from the Affordable Care Act) were released by the Departments of Treasury, Labor and Health and Human Services for public comment.[32] Comments were due by January 25, 2013. The proposed regulations include 16 significant revisions to the statute, two of which impact the approach proposed in Appendix A. The expectation is that at least one more revision and probably two will be released based on comments submitted. The final regulations are expected to be released by January 1, 2014, because all provisions in the statue will be in effect on that date. Employers should develop programs based on the provisions in the statute until the final regulations are released.

Participation in programs being sufficient for the full discount

The proposed regulations recommend that employees who do not meet health standards, eg. they use tobacco, are overweight, etc., be able to qualify for the health standard and receive the full premium discount by participating in a wellness program to help them meet the standard. This revision to the statute eviscerates the concept of different levels of rewards for participating in programs versus meeting the health standard. This change was opposed by most employer groups and supported by some patient advocate groups. If this rule is retained in the final regulations, the approach described in Appendix A would need to be modified to eliminate the different levels of discount for meeting the health standard versus participating in a program.

Maximum discount increased from 30% to 50%

The proposed regulations recommend that the maximum discount in effect on January 1, 2014, be increased from 30% to 50% on the condition that one of the health standards is being tobacco free. As such, the maximum discount for meeting all other health standards would be 30%, thus allowing 20% for being tobacco free. The statute in the Affordable Care Act allows a maximum discount of 20% until January 1, 2014, specifies that the maximum will increase to at least 30% on that date, and gives the Secretaries of Treasury and Health and Human Services the authority to increase the maximum to 50% on that date. Reactions to this proposed rule were mixed, with no clear pattern of supporters and opponents, and many not commenting. In the author's opinion, the 50% level discount is not necessary from a motivation perspective, so the recommended approach would not need to be modified from what is described in Appendix A. Also, given the fact that few employers offer discounts at the 20% range now permitted, it is unlikely that most employers will increase the discount to the full 50%. However, if the 50% maximum is retained, some employers are likely to increase to the maximum and that the overall average discount among all employers is likely to increase.

Appendix C

Vendor Savings Guarantees

By Steven P. Noeldner, PhD, Partner, Mercer Health & Benefits, LLC

I. Introduction

In the early 2000s, disease management/medical condition management providers started offering employers guarantees that their programs would save money in excess of their costs. In recent years, health promotion providers have started to offer similar savings guarantees. There are no known surveys on the prevalence of savings guarantee agreements, however, they seem to be common among 1) large national providers who offer comprehensive health promotion programs that are expected to improve or eliminate health risk factors and reduce medical care costs[33] and 2) very large self-insured employers (i.e. 3,000 or more employees). They are most common when the health promotion provider is a health insurance carrier or a national vendor and when a consultant releases a national request for proposal (RFP) on behalf of the employer and includes the savings guarantee as a preferred element of the RFP. Savings guarantees are sometimes offered to medium sized employers (1,000 to 2,999 employees), and sometimes by regional health promotion providers, but not very often. Savings guarantees are rarely, if ever, offered by providers who specialize in individual program components, such as health risk assessments, screening programs, individual behavior change programs, fitness center management, and other limited services; or when the employer is small, fully- insured and/or is part of a pooled health insurance group.

II. Structure of Agreements
A. Risk and Flow of Payments

It is common for health promotion providers that offer savings guarantees to put at risk some financial stake, typically a percentage of the fees they charge, to support the savings guarantee to their clients. The amount of the financial stake varies considerably depending upon such factors as the amount of program fees collected by the vendor, whether or not the vendor is competing with other vendors for the business, and the negotiating skills of the employer or consultant representing the employer. When providers offer savings guarantees with some of their fees at risk, they typically build additional revenue into their fee structure to cover their financial risk. Some vendors may increase their service fees to the employer by an amount equivalent to their fees at risk, while others may only increase fees by a fraction of their fees at risk. The magnitude of the increase in service fees may also be influenced by the provider's perception of how its fees will compare to those of competitors vying for the client's business.

In one common model for a medical cost savings guarantee, the health promotion provider and employer agree on a fixed percentage of the annual program fees that will be refunded to the employer if the cost savings for the program do not meet or exceed agreed upon targets. For example, savings targets may be expressed in terms of Return on Investment (ROI) and set at 0.8:1 for the first program year, 1.5:1 for the second program year, and 2:1 for the third program year. The percent of service fees that is eligible for refund may, for example, start at 5% in year one and increase in the second and third years. This is consistent with the idea that as health promotion programs mature, greater cost savings are expected and more weight (greater fees at risk) is placed on savings as a program outcome. If the provider builds extra revenue into its service fees to cover the savings guarantee, then when savings targets are met, the excess fees are retained by the provider as additional profit.

Another relatively new, but emerging approach is gain-sharing. In this model, the provider and employer agree in advance on a savings calculation methodology and on the proportions of savings attributed to the health promotion program the employer and provider will share. One example of a gain-sharing split might be 30% to the provider with 70% retained by the employer. In this arrangement, the employer would pay the provider its share of the cost savings (gain) after the program period (typically annually). Gain-sharing would be in lieu of a provider raising its service fees to cover fees it puts at risk for achieving a savings target.

B. Employer Requirements

Providers that offer savings guarantees often require the employer to agree to a number of conditions. A multi-year contract, typically a minimum of three years, is common. A variety of implementation elements may be required of the employer as well, such as having a structured communication plan, incentives for employees to participate, a high percentage of accurate contact information, and in some cases, a minimum participation rate (although employers may expect the provider to be responsible for participation rates if the employer is providing incentives and promotional support).

C. Evaluation Methodology

There are a number of factors that should be considered when a savings guarantee is established. The methodology used to calculate cost savings will determine how precise – and believable – the outcome will be. The methodology selected should also dictate the savings target. Robust methodologies that control for confounding influences typically yield more precise (and often more conservative) results compared to methodologies that predict or estimate cost savings.

Selecting an appropriate evaluation methodology on which both provider and employer agree is an important first step. A variety of factors should be considered, including what type of data is available (e.g., health care claims data, time-over-time health risk assessment results for the same individuals, etc.), the number of program participants, and the evaluation resources available to the provider or employer (e.g., capable evaluation staff, statistical analysis technology, funding, etc.).

Health Risk Assessment (HRA) Data. Wellness or lifestyle management program providers historically have utilized individual-level HRA data from participants who completed the HRA both at the beginning and the end of an evaluation period (e.g., program year) to estimate health care cost savings for risk factors that have been reduced or eliminated. Most "predictive" methodologies have been developed using health care costs associated with individual health risk factors as reported in the landmark Health Enhancement Research Organization (HERO) studies near the end of the 1990s.[34, 35]

While these predictive methodologies are useful and may provide good directional estimates of program cost savings, they are subject to a number of challenges to their precision. For example, how the estimated cost savings for any individual health risk factor is allocated over time – e.g., assigning some portion of the total cost savings in the first year a health risk was eliminated, compared to assigning portions of the total cost savings over a number of years – could influence the magnitude of the ascribed savings in any one program year.

Health Care Claims Data. The use of actual medical and pharmacy claims data is far superior to costs tied to proxy measures such as self-reported health habits. As such, a growing number of health promotion providers are now using claims data to evaluate cost savings.

Trend Analysis vs. Matched Controls. Even when individual-level health care claims data are available, there are different approaches to determining cost savings. Until recently, some form of health care cost trend analysis was often utilized to calculate cost savings, or more precisely, cost avoidance for those who participated in a health promotion program.

Trend analysis typically compares the employer's health care cost experience prior to the implementation of a health promotion program to its cost experience after the program has been in place for a year or more. The difference between the "expected" trend that might have occurred if no program had been implemented, and the "actual" health care costs measured during the evaluation period, is assumed to be associated with the impact of the health promotion program.

While trend analysis may appear to be an attractive methodology, it is subject to a number of potentially confounding influences. Factors that can influence the accuracy of the results of the trend methodology include differences from base line to intervention period in health plan design (e.g., cost sharing, mix of plan types offered, provider networks, etc.), health plan carrier (if it changed), and composition of the employee population (e.g., healthier employees are added to the workforce, less healthy employees depart).

A more robust alternative to the health care cost trend analysis is the matched-control, multivariate regression analysis methodology, which typically yields a more precise (and conservative) analysis of health care cost savings associated with health promotion program participation. This is a claims-based, multi-step methodology which first uses statistical techniques to find close matches between program participants and non-participants (controls). Some factors typically used for matching include age, gender, health status (or risk score), and health care costs. After a closely-matched control group is identified, the difference in costs for participants from the baseline period (prior to the program) to the end of the evaluation period (at least one program year) is compared to the difference in cost for controls from baseline to the end of evaluation period. This "difference-in-difference" value is considered the cost savings associated with program participation.

D. Savings Targets

The amount of the savings target will be influenced both by the quality of the program and evaluation methodology. In the author's experience, less precise predictive or estimation methodologies sometimes result in higher savings values than those calculated using more rigorous matched-control regression analysis. Because of the potential for numerous confounding influences when using the trend-based methodology, calculated savings using this methodology are typically higher than when using the matched-control regression analysis methodology. Similarly, predictive methodologies that assign a savings value to reduced or eliminated health risks, often provide inflated estimates of true cost savings and should have savings targets adjusted accordingly. This trend is not consistent with the published literature. For example, in a meta-analysis involving 22 studies on the impact of health promotion programs on medical care costs, the studies with randomized experimental designs had ROIs averaging 3.36, while those with non-randomized designs had ROIs of 2.38.[36]

E. Evaluator

Most cost savings evaluations are done by the vendors that provide the health promotion programs. Rarely does the employer conduct the analysis, primarily because it lacks the necessary expertise or resources. On occasion, larger employers that have made substantial investments for their health promotion programs, engage a third-party evaluator, usually a data analysis or consulting firm. When a third-party is the evaluator, the methodology used is typically a more robust, matched-control regression analysis.

III. Challenges, Risks and Opportunities

Accurate measurement of health care cost savings associated with health promotion programs is a challenging endeavor. The resources required to gather and analyze data are considerable. Most employers and vendors don't have adequate expertise to conduct a robust savings analysis, and the considerable cost of an analysis can erode savings generated by the program. Typically, only employers that have invested substantially in their programs, or expect very large gross savings amounts, will pay for a robust savings analysis to verify their program's financial outcomes.

One notable threat to the successful utilization of savings guarantee agreements is the potentially adversarial relationship it may establish and foster. If the employer has an opportunity to be refunded some of its program fees if the vendor misses the savings target, it may not be fully motivated to provide the support needed for the program to succeed. Conversely, if the vendor has fee revenue or a portion of a gain-share at stake, it may be motivated to utilize an imprecise evaluation methodology, or even falsify or skew the interpretation of results to avoid refunding fees, or to achieve a greater "gain".

If an employer can justify the expense of a precise cost savings evaluation using a robust methodology (ideally conducted by a qualified third party), a gain-sharing arrangement with the vendor may establish the most positive and productive employer-vendor relationship. Gain-sharing can motivate both employer and vendor to do all they can, separately and collectively, to assure the success of health promotion programs. If the employer is unable or unwilling to commit the resources needed to conduct a robust savings analysis, it may be reasonable to forgo a savings guarantee to avoid higher vendor service fees to cover the vendor's fees at risk for the savings guarantee.

IV. Recommended Approach

The following approach may be used to support decision-making about the appropriateness and approach to savings guarantees.

1. Decide if a savings guarantee is desired by the employer and acceptable to the vendor.

2. If yes, review the skill level available to design and execute the study and the quality of data available.
3. Develop a study methodology that matches the skill level, available data and the financial terms of the guarantee, as well as protocols to resolve disagreements.
4. Confirm the party responsible for each element of the study methodology.

Appendix D

HERO Scorecard and CDC Scorecard

HERO Scorecard

The HERO Best Practice Scorecard© was developed as a tool to help employers improve the quality of their health promotion programs by documenting program components, primarily from a management perspective. The Scorecard can be used as an inventory to catalogue a program's components, an indicator of success in implementing program components and as a comparative benchmarking tool to compare a program with peer employers. HERO has published several reports summarizing findings drawn from the database of responses.

In version 3.1, the core questionnaire has 62 questions organized into six major sections: strategic planning (10 questions), leadership engagement (6 questions), program level management (8 questions), programs (22 questions), engagement methods (13 questions), and measurement and evaluation (3 questions). It also has an optional section on outcomes, with more detailed questions on participation rates in the various program areas, program costs, and impact of programs on health risks and medical costs.

The Scorecard was developed through a collaborative process involving several dozen leading authorities in health promotion who volunteered their time and expertise to HERO (Health Enhancement Research Organization), and Mercer who provided expertise in health promotion and technical support to produce the tools. The first edition was developed in 2006. Version 3.1 was released in March of 2012 and version 4 was in development at the time this book was published. More details can be found at HERO Scorecard website:[37] http://www.the-hero.org

After completing the Scorecard online a report is sent to the user showing the score for their organization and average scores for all other organizations. The Scorecard and a follow-up report with scores for the individual user organization and average aggregate scores for all other organization users are provided at no charge to all users. More detailed reports with aggregated responses for each question, breakdowns of scores by industry, geographic region, and employer size can be purchased.

The CDC Worksite Health ScoreCard: An Assessment Tool for Employers to Prevent Heart Disease, Stroke, & Related Health Conditions

The CDC Worksite Health ScoreCard[38] was developed to help employers determine if they have implemented evidence based interventions and strategies. It focuses primarily on the components of individual program interventions but includes a short section on organization level design.

The questionnaire contains 100 questions that assess the extent to which evidence-based strategies have been used in programs. The strategies include counseling services, environmental supports, policies, health plan benefits, and other worksite programs shown to be effective in preventing heart disease, stroke, and related health conditions. The 100 questions are organized into 12 major sections: organizational supports (18 questions), tobacco control (10 questions), nutrition (13 questions), physical activity (9 questions), weight management (5 questions), stress management (6 questions), depression (7 questions), high blood pressure (7 questions), high cholesterol (6 questions), diabetes (6 questions), signs and symptoms of heart attack and stroke (4 questions) and emergency response to heart attack and stroke (9 questions). Users tally their own scores manually and there is no mechanism to add scores to a central database.

All of the items in the questionnaire are tied to strategies that have been documented in the scientific literature to be effective. From a scoring perspective, the relative value of each item is weighted to reflect both the magnitude of impact of the approach and the quality of published evidence supporting its impact. References to the scientific literature are provided for each topic area. The questionnaire was field tested with a sample of 93 very small, small, medium, and large worksites for validity and reliability, and feasibility of adopting the strategies highlighted in the tool.

The Appendix of the Scorecard includes an example of the strategies, processes, communications and evaluation elements that might be in a plan to achieve several specific health goals. It also includes sample program budgets, and blank templates that can be used to prepare plans and budgets.

The CDC Scorecard was developed by a team of professionals at CDC and Emory University. It was released in September of 2012. More information can be found at The Worksite Health Scorecard website: http://www.cdc.gov/dhdsp/pubs/worksite_scorecard.htm

References

1   O'Donnell MP. Definition of Health Promotion 2.0: Embracing Passion, Enhancing Motivation, Recognizing Dynamic Balance, and Creating Opportunities. *Amer J Health Promot.* 2009;24:iv–iv.

2   O'Donnell M, Bishop C, Kaplan K. Benchmarking best practices in workplace health promotion programs. *Am J Health Promot.* 1997;1:TAHP-1-8.

3   Linnan L, Bowling M, Childress J, Lindsay G, et al. Results of the 2004 National Worksite Health Promotion Survey. *Am J Public Health.* 2008;98:1503-9.

4   Gould L, Ornish D, Scher W, Brown S, et al. Changes in myocardial perfusion abnormalities by positron emission tomography after long-term, intense risk factor modification. *JAMA.* 1995;274:894-901.

5   Prochaska J, Velicer W. The transtheoretical model of health behavior change. *Am J Health Promot.* 1997;12:38-48.

6   O'Donnell M. Health impact of workplace health promotion programs and methodological quality of the research literature. *Am J Health Promot.* 1997;1:TAHP-1-8.

7   Heaney C, Goetzel R. A review of health related outcomes of multi-component workplace health promotion programs. *Am J Health Promot.* 1997;11:290-307.

8   U.S. Department of Health and Human Services. Clinical Practice Guideline: Treating Tobacco Use and Dependence: 2008 Update. Available at: http://www.surgeongeneral.gov/tobacco/treating_tobacco_use08.pdf. Accessed August 23, 2012.

9   Seaverson ELD, Grossmeier J, Miller TM, Anderson DA. The role of incentive design, incentive value, communications strategy, and worksite culture on health risk assessment participation. *Am J Health Promot.* 2009;23:343-52.

10 Taitel MS, Haufle V, Heck D, Loeppke R, Fetterolf D. Incentives and other factors associated with employee participation in health risk assessment. *J Occup Environ Med.* 2008;50:863–872.

11 Matson D, Lee J, Hopp J. The impact of incentives and competitions on participation and quit rates in worksite smoking cessation programs. *Am J Health Promot.* 1993;7:270-280.

12 Baicker K, Cutler D, Song Z. Workplace Wellness Programs Can Generate Savings. *Health Aff.* 2010;29:304-311.

13 Chapman LS. Meta-Evaluation of Worksite Health Promotion Economic Return Studies: 2012 Update. *Am J Health Promot.* 2012;26:TAHP-1-TAHP-12.

14 Baicker K, Cutler D, Song Z, Workplace Wellness Programs Can Generate Savings, Health Affairs, 29, no. 2 (2010): 304-311.

15 Towers Watson. 2011/2012 Staying@Work Survey Report: A Pathway to Employee Health and Workplace Productivity. Available at: http://www.towerswatson.com/united-states/research/6031. Accessed August 16, 2012.

16 Incentives for Nondiscriminatory Wellness Programs in Group Health Plans, Federal Register, Vol 78, No. 106, June 3, 2013. Available at: https://www.federalregister.gov/articles/2013/06/03/2013-12916/incentives-for-nondiscriminatory-wellness-programs-in-group-health-plans. Accessed June 12, 2013.

17 Taitel, M. S., V. Haufle, D. Heck, et al. Incentives and other factors associated with employee participation in health risk assessment. *J Occup Environ Med* 2008. 50:863–872.

18 Seaverson, E. L. D., J. Grossmeier, T. M. Miller, and D. A. Anderson. The role of incentive design, incentive, value, communications strategy, and worksite culture on health risk assessment participation. *Am J Health Promot* 2009. 23:343.

19 Goetzel RZ, Anderson DR, Whitmer RW, Ozminkowski RJ, et al. The relationship between modifiable health risks and health care expenditures: an analysis of the multi-employer HERO health risk and cost database. *J Occup Environ Med.* 1998;40:843–854.

20 ACLU briefing paper 12.The 'Lectric Law Library site. Available at: http://www.lectlaw.com/files/emp08.htm. Accessed August 24, 2012.

21 Secondhand Smoke (SHS) Facts. Centers for Disease Control and Prevention site. Available at: http://www.cdc.gov/tobacco/data_statistics/fact_sheets /secondhand_smoke/general_facts/. Accessed August 18, 2010.

22 Centers for Disease Control and Prevention (CDC).Cigarette smoking-attributable morbidity—United States, 2000.*MMWR Morb Mortal Wkly Rep.* 2003;52:842–844.

23 McClave AK, Whitney N, Thorne SL, Mariolis P, et al. Adult tobacco survey—19 States, 2003–2007. *MMWR SurveillSumm.* 2010;59:1–75

24 Centers for Disease Control and Prevention (CDC). Annual smoking-attributable mortality, years of potential life lost, and economic costs–United States, 1995-1999. *MMWR Morb Mortal Wkly Rep.* 2002;51:300-3.

25 O'Donnell MP, Roizen MF. The SmokingPaST Framework: Illustrating the Impact of Quit Attempts, Quit Methods, and New Smokers on Smoking Prevalence, Years of Life Saved, Medical Costs Saved, Programming Costs, Cost Effectiveness, and Return on Investment. *Am J Health Promot.* 2011;26:e11-e23.

26 State Smoker Protection Laws. American Lung Association site. Available at: http://www.lungusa2.org/slati/appendixf.php. Accessed August 24, 2012.

27 Linnan L, Bowling M, Childress J, Lindsay G. Results of the 2004 National Worksite Health Promotion Survey. *Am J Public Health.* 2008;98:1503-9.

28 Henry J. Kaiser Family Foundation, Health Research and Educational Trust. Employer Health Benefits 2011 Annual Survey. Kaiser Family Foundation site. Available at: http://ehbs.kff.org/pdf/2011/8225. pdf. Accessed August 24, 2012

29 C. Everett Koop National Health Award. The Health Project site. Available at: http://www.thehealthproject. com/index.html. Accessed August 23, 2012.

30 Sui X, LaMonte MJ, Laditka JN, Hardin JW, et al. Cardiorespiratory fitness and adiposity as mortality predictors in older adults. *JAMA.* 2007;298:2507–2516.

31 O'Donnell MP. Making the Impossible Possible: Engaging the Entire Population in Comprehensive Workplace Health Promotion Programs at No Net Cost to Employers or Employees. *Am J Health Promot.* 2010;24:iv-v.

32 Incentives for Nondiscriminatory Wellness Programs in Group Health Plans. Federal Register / Vol. 77, No. 227 / Monday, November 26, 2012 / Proposed Rules. 70620-70642.

33 Serxner S, Gold D, Meraz A, Gray A. Do employee health management programs work? *Amer J Health Promot.* 2009;23:TAHP-1-8,iii.

34 Anderson DR, Whitmer RW, Goetzel RZ, Ozminkowski JR, et al. The relationship between modifiable health risks and group-level health care expenditures. *Amer J Health Promot.* 2000;15:45-52.

35 Goetzel, R.Z., Anderson, D.R., Whitmer, R.W., Ozminkowski, J.R., Dunn, R.L., Wasserman, J., HERO Research Committee (1998). The relationship between modifiable health risks and health care expenditures. *Journal of Occupational and Environmental Medicine,* 40(10), 1-12.

36 HERO Best Practice Scorecard in Collaboration with Mercer. The Health Enhancement Research Organization site. Available at: http://www.the-hero.org/scorecard_folder/scorecard.htm. Accessed September 11, 2012.

37 Centers for Disease Control and Prevention. *The CDC Worksite Health ScoreCard: An Assessment Tool for Employers to Prevent Heart Disease, Stroke, and Related Health Conditions.* Available at: http://www.cdc.gov/dhdsp/pubs/worksite_scorecard.htm. Accessed September 11, 2012.

38 Baicker K, Cutler D, Song Z. Workplace wellness programs can generate savings. Health Aff (Millwood). 2010 Feb;29(2):304-11. Epub 2010 Jan 14.

About the Author

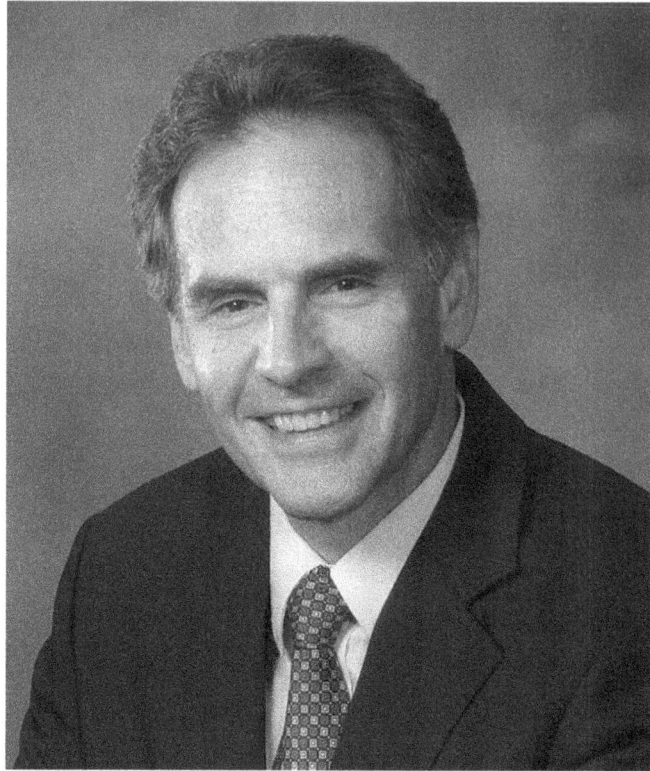

Dr. O'Donnell is the Director of the Health Management Research Center in the School of Kinesiology of the University of Michigan. Formed in 1978, the Center has helped more than 1000 worksites measure the health risks of their employees; calculate the link between health risks, medical costs and productivity; evaluate the impact of their health promotion programs; and in the process, establish the scientific foundation for this area of research. Dr. O'Donnell has worked directly with employers, health care organizations, government agencies, foundations, insurance companies and health promotion providers to develop new and refine existing health promotion programs and has served in leadership roles in four major health systems. He is Founder, President and Editor-in-Chief of the *American Journal of Health Promotion* and is also Founder and Chairman Emeritus of Health Promotion Advocates, a non-profit policy group created to integrate health promotion strategies into national policy. Health Promotion Advocates was successful in developing six provisions that became law as part of the Affordable Care Act. He has co-authored 6 books and workbooks, including *Health Promotion in the Workplace,* which was in continuous publication for 27 years, and more than 190 articles, book chapters and columns. He has presented more than 260 keynote and workshop presentations on six continents, served on boards and committees for 48 non-profit and for-profit organizations and received 13 national awards. His most recent awards are the Elizabeth Fries Health Education Award presented by the James F. and Sarah T. Fries Foundation, and the Bill Whitmer Leadership Award, presented by the Health Enhancement Research Organization (HERO). He earned a PhD in Health Behavior from University of Michigan, an MBA in General Management and an MPH in Hospital Management, both from University of California, Berkeley, and an AB in psychobiology from Oberlin College. He attended high school and was later a Senior Fulbright Scholar and visiting professor in Seoul, Korea.